The
Medical
Transcriptionist's
Guide

to

Microsoft Word®

Third Edition
Make It Your Own
Workbook

The
Medical
Transcriptionist's
Guide

to
Microsoft Word®

Third Edition
Make It Your Own
Workbook

Laura Bryan MT (ASCP), CMT

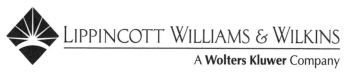

LIPPINCOTT WILLIAMS & WILKINS
A **Wolters Kluwer** Company

Philadelphia · Baltimore · New York · London
Buenos Aires · Hong Kong · Sydney · Tokyo

www.makeityourown.stedmans.com

Publisher: Julie Stegman
Managing Editor: Lisa Manhart
Production Coordinator: Jason Delaney
Typesetter: Maryland Composition, Inc.
Printer & Binder: Quebecor World-Taunton

Copyright © 2005 Lippincott Williams & Wilkins
351 West Camden Street
Baltimore, Maryland 21201-2436

Printed in the United States of America

Contents

Preface

This workbook is written specifically to accompany the *Medical Transcriptionist's Guide to Microsoft Word®, 3rd Edition* and is designed to give the transcriptionist, whether a "newbie" or a veteran, a structured approach to learning Microsoft Word® for medical transcription. The questions emphasize concepts that are especially important for transcription, and the majority of the questions require an explanation, as this encourages the student to study the material and then formulate an answer. My intention is to show MTs how to *apply* Microsoft Word® to their daily tasks in order to improve production and accuracy, not just how to *use* Word to type. As many transcriptionists will tell you, "the money is in the keyboard," and keeping your hands on the keys increases production, so there is also a special emphasis on shortcut keys and keyboarding skills. Troubleshooting issues are also covered, including ways to locate files, recover files after a shutdown, and how to backup important data including shortcuts and macros.

The first three lessons cover basic concepts for navigating through the Windows environment and also managing files and folders. The fourth lesson introduces the Word interface and the many elements displayed on the screen when Word is running. Formatting is covered extensively in lesson five, followed by templates and fields in lesson six. The productivity-enhancing features—AutoCorrect, AutoText, and Macros—are covered together in lesson seven in order to compare and contrast the three. Questions are designed to help the transcriptionist determine how and when to apply each feature. Editing is becoming a large part of transcription and is expected to increase as voice recognition is used more extensively, so lesson eight focuses on shortcut keys for quickly navigating and editing a document and also techniques for the QA editor. Lesson nine concentrates on basic skills for customizing Word.

Lessons 1–9 include a reading assignment taken from the *Medical Transcriptionist's Guide to Microsft Word®, 3rd Edition* and one or more video presentations taken from the CD that accompanies the *Guide.* Each lesson includes objective questions with answers in the

Answer Key at the back of the workbook. In addition, each lesson includes hands-on exercises for practice. There are no answers provided for the exercises, as they are intended to help the student put into practice the skills and concepts covered in each lesson. Instructors who would like their students to document these exercises may use the "Print Screen" method explained on page 241 of the *Guide*.

Lesson ten is an exercise in problem solving. The scenarios presented are those commonly encountered by transcriptionists using MS Word. The Answer Key gives the page number of the *Guide* where the solution may be found.

It is my sincere hope that you will have many "aha" moments as you work through these lessons. Finding new and clever ways to work can be fun, especially when it translates to less frustration and, of course, more income! Think of each lesson as "money in the bank" and you will find yourself smiling all the way through the book.

—Laura Bryan, CMT
February 2005

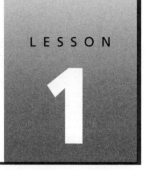

Windows Elements and Shortcut Keys

INTRODUCTION

This first lesson will introduce basic keyboarding concepts in Windows as well as universal shortcut keys. Using the keyboard and shortcut keys is the best way to work more efficiently whether you are working in Word or Windows.

Objectives:

1. Identify common Windows elements
2. Understand keyboarding concepts
3. Use Universal shortcut keys
4. Use the Logo Key

READ AND WATCH

Chapter 1, pp 3–12, Appendix A, Glossary

Introduction to Windows

TEST YOUR KNOWLEDGE

Answer the following questions:

1. Explain the difference between commands written with a plus sign (ALT+D) and commands written with a comma (ALT, D).

_____

_____

2. How are hot keys identified?

_____

_____

3. What is an alpha character?

_____

_____

4. Give the definition of a menu.

_____

_____

5. Explain how to open any menu in Windows.

_____

_____

6. Name two functions of the Title bar.

_____

_____

7. How do you minimize any program using the keyboard?

_____

_____

8. Which key will open the Start menu?

_____

_____

9. Which shortcut key combination will open Windows Explorer?

_____

_____

10. Which shortcut key combination will minimize all open
applications and take you to the Windows Desktop?

_____

_____

11. What is the purpose of the Taskbar?

_____

_____

12. Which key will always take you to the beginning of a
line of text? To the end of a line of text?

_____

_____

13. Explain Cut, Copy, and Paste.

_____

_____

_____

14. What is the shortcut key combination to select all?

_____

_____

15. What is the universal shortcut key for renaming a folder?

_____

_____

16. Which key will take you back to the previous folder level
or previous web page?

_____

_____

17. What do the + and − signs mean in a file tree?

_____

_____

18. How do you select a drive or folder in a file tree using
     the keyboard?

_____

_____

19. Define a dialogue box.

_____

_____

20. Describe two ways to move the cursor inside a dialogue
     box using the keyboard.

_____

_____

21. List two possible ways to move between tabs in a
     dialogue box using the keyboard.

_____

_____

22. Which key will place or remove a check mark or select a
     radio button in a dialogue box?

_____

_____

23. How is the cursor location indicated in a dialogue box?

_____

_____

24. How do you close a dialogue box or cancel an action?

_____

_____

Give the command for these shortcut keys:

25. ALT+F4   _____

26. ALT+Tab   _____

27. CTRL+C   _____

28. CTRL+V   _____

29. CTRL+X   _____

30. F3   _____

31. F1   _____

32. F4   _____

33. Esc   _____

34. F6   _____

35. Logo+F   _____

36. ALT or F10   _____

37. Logo+Pause/break   _____

38. CTRL+ALT+Del   _____

Fill in the blanks:

39. Using Figure 1-2, on page 7 of the workbook, give the name of the folder that is open.

_____

_____

40. What View is shown in Figure 1-2 on page 7 of the workbook?

_____

_____

APPLY YOUR SKILLS

41. Label Figure 1-1 with the following items:

The Desktop

The Start Menu

The lower part of the Start Menu

The upper part of the Start Menu

An icon

The Taskbar

The QuickLaunch bar

The Notification Area/System Tray

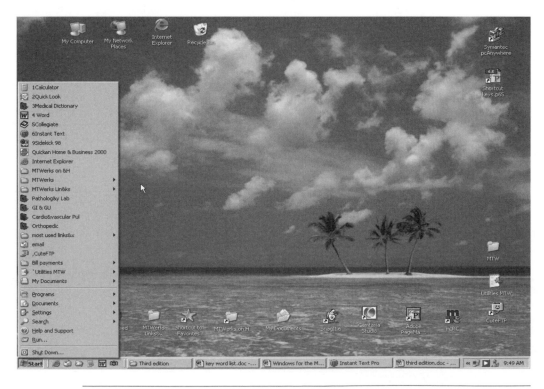

FIGURE 1-1

42.   Label Figure 1-2 with the following items:

The Menu bar

The Title bar

The Address bar

Shortcut menu

Hot key

Toolbar

Explorer bar

Border for resizing

Scroll bar

File list area

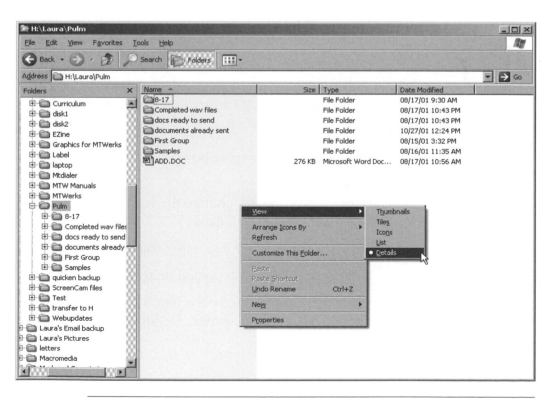

FIGURE 1-2

43. Using the directions on page 249 of the *Guide*, fill in the following information from your own computer.

   Version of your operating
   system   _____

   System name   _____

   User name   _____

   Version of Word   _____

44. Use the keyboard to step through the following:

   a. Open Windows Explorer, Word, and one other program of your choice.

   b. Minimize all three windows using Logo+D.

   c. Use ALT+Tab to make Word the active window.

   d. Use the keyboard to minimize Word.

   e. Use ATL+Tab to make the Explorer window active.

   f. Use the keyboard to open the View menu on the Explorer window and change the View to Details.

   g. Use ALT+F4 to close all three windows.

45. Use the keyboard to step through the following:

   a. Open Word.

   b. Open the Font dialogue box using the shortcut CTRL+D.

   c. Using the keyboard, change the font settings to Courier New, Italic, 12 pt., all caps.

   d. Type several lines of text using the above font settings.

   e. Select the text you just typed using CTRL+A.

   f. Open the Font dialogue box again and change the font back to Times New Roman, Regular, 10 pt., not all caps.

g. Press CTRL+S to save the document. Give the file a name such as Exercise B. Save the document in the folder called My Documents.

h. Close Word (using the File menu command and the keyboard).

i. Open Explorer and use the keyboard to navigate to My Documents. Locate the file just created. Use the shortcut key combination to copy the file.

j. Open any other folder and use the shortcut command to paste a copy of Exercise B.doc into that folder.

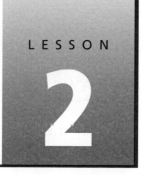

Mouse Techniques and Shortcut Icons

INTRODUCTION

While the keyboard is quite helpful for improving efficiency, there are still a few mouse tricks that help get the job done quickly and easily. This lesson focuses on several mouse techniques including those that combine the left and right mouse buttons with keyboard keys to expand the mouse's capability. Also included in this discussion are "context sensitive" menus, also called right-click menus. In the last part of this lesson, you will learn how to take full advantage of shortcut icons.

Objectives:

1. Use various mouse techniques
2. Use right-click menus
3. Create and use shortcut icons

READ AND WATCH

 Chapter 2, pp 15–24, Appendix A, pp 254–256, Glossary

 Create shortcuts in Windows
Create shortcuts on the Start Menu

TEST YOUR KNOWLEDGE

Answer the following questions:

1. Define context sensitive menus.

   _____

   _____

2. What is an "object?"

   _____

   _____

3. In Windows, Properties refers to:

   _____

   _____

4. How do you access Display Properties from the Desktop?

   _____

   _____

5. Explain how to tile windows horizontally.

   _____

   _____

6. How do you learn about an option or command in a dialogue box?

   _____

   _____

7. List at least three commands you might find on the shortcut menu when you right-click on a file name.

   _____

   _____

8. What can you do using the Send to menu?

9. What happens if you right-click a shortcut icon and choose Send to/Mail recipient?

10. Does the Send to menu command copy the file or move the file?

11. Which key on the keyboard is the same as a right-click?

12. How are shortcut icons distinguished from other icons?

13. Does a shortcut icon affect the location of the file, folder, or application?

14. Does the shortcut name have to be the same as the file or folder name?

15. How many shortcuts can you place on the Start (Main) menu?

_____

_____

16. Define Drag and Drop.

_____

_____

_____

17. Explain Shift+Click and CTRL+Click.

_____

_____

_____

18. Explain CTRL+Drag and ALT+Drag.

_____

_____

_____

Identify these icons:

19. ⬉   _____

20. ⬉?   _____

21. +   _____

22. ↔   _____

23.   ⊕   _____

24.   👆   _____

APPLY YOUR SKILLS

25.   Step through the following:

   a. Create a shortcut to your favorite web site and place it on the Desktop.

   b. Rename the shortcut you just created using the right-click menu.

   c. Using Explorer, locate a file or folder that you use frequently. Right-click on the file or folder and create a shortcut on the Desktop.

   d. Choose a shortcut on your Desktop and drag it to the Start menu.

   e. Rename the shortcut so that the shortcut name starts with a unique character.

   f. Open the file or folder using the Logo key and the hot key for that shortcut.

26.   Step through the following:

   a. Open Word.

   b. Type a paragraph of text, purposely misspelling several words and leaving out commas or periods.

   c. Right-click on the misspelled words using the Application key and correct the spelling using the Arrow keys and the Enter key to select the correct word.

   d. Right-click on the grammatical errors (marked with a wavy green line) and correct the grammar. Do this without using the mouse.

27. Step through the following:

   a. If you are using Windows XP, follow the instructions on page 23 of the *Guide* to change your Start menu to Classic Style. (Change it back if you prefer the double-column style.)

   b. Follow the directions on page 24 of the *Guide* for using small icons on the Start menu. (Change the setting back to large icons if you prefer.)

28. Step through the following:

   a. Open Word.

   b. Open WordPad (Start>Programs>Accessories>WordPad).

   c. Right-click on the Taskbar and choose Tile windows vertically.

   d. Type a paragraph in the Word window.

   e. Press CTRL+A to select all of the text.

   f. Press CTRL+C to copy the selected text.

   g. Use ALT+Tab to change the focus from Word to WordPad.

   h. Press CTRL+V to paste the text into WordPad.

   i. Use ALT+Tab to make Word the active application.

   j. If the text is no longer selected, use CTRL+A to select the text again.

   k. Use the drag and drop technique to drag the selected text from Word to WordPad. Notice the mouse cursor will change and have a + sign attached to it.

29. Step through the following:

   a. Right-click on the Taskbar and choose Properties.

   b. Right-click on each option, choose "What's This?" and read the description.

Files, Folders, and Security

INTRODUCTION

This lesson will cover important concepts in Windows, including files and folders and how to manage them using Windows Explorer and the Save As and Open dialogue boxes. In addition, you will learn how to locate files and folders using Windows Search (also called Find). The lesson will finish up with ways to protect files while you transcribe and how to back up critical files for running MS Word.

Objectives:

1. Recognize common file extensions
2. Use Folders
3. Use Windows Explorer
4. Use the Save As and Open dialogue boxes
5. Use Windows Search
6. Safeguard data and files

READ AND WATCH

 Chapter 3, pp 25–43

 Change the Default Working Folder
Create a Backup Routine

TEST YOUR KNOWLEDGE

Answer the following questions:

1. Define file extension.

   _____

   _____

2. List three examples of file extensions and their associations.

   _____

   _____

3. Define folder.

   _____

   _____

4. How many folders can you create (i.e., what is the limit)?

   _____

   _____

5. What is contained in a System folder?

   _____

   _____

6. Define path name.

   _____

   _____

7. What is the difference between an address (path name) that starts with backslash (\) and one that starts with two forward slashes (//)?

   _____

   _____

8. What is Windows Explorer?

   _____

   _____

9. Can you open more than one copy of Windows Explorer?

   _____

   _____

10. Name at least three tasks you can perform using the Open and Save As dialogue boxes.

    _____

    _____

11. The Open and Save As dialogue boxes automatically open with which folder selected?

    _____

    _____

12. Using the keyboard, how do you move from the File name box to the File list area in the Save As dialogue box?

    _____

    _____

13. How do you sort a list of files in the Open or Save As dialogue boxes?

    _____

    _____

14. List at least three ways of displaying the contents of a folder.

    _____

    _____

15. What is contained in the Favorites folder?

_____

_____

16. Define browsing.

_____

_____

17. How do you find hidden files?

_____

_____

_____

18. What information do you need in order to search for a file or folder?

_____

_____

19. List two boolean characters and what they mean.

_____

_____

20. Name five things you can do once you locate a file using Windows Search.

_____

_____

21. List three of Word's program files that should be backed up on a regular basis.

_____

_____

22. What is the best way to safeguard your work *while* still transcribing the document?

_____

_____

23. What two things are required in order for AutoRecover to work?

_____

_____

24. Explain how to restore a document after a shutdown using AutoRecover.

_____

_____

_____

25. If Word is forced to close improperly, what should you do to make sure there are no remnants of Word left open?

_____

_____

Match-up the following icons:

These icons were taken from the Save As dialogue box. Match the icon to its corresponding command.

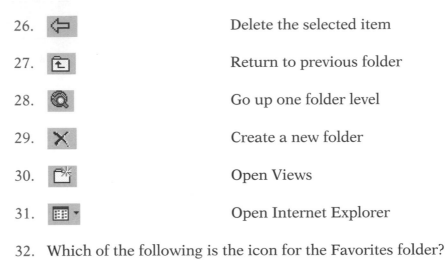

26.   Delete the selected item

27.   Return to previous folder

28.   Go up one folder level

29.   Create a new folder

30.   Open Views

31.   Open Internet Explorer

32. Which of the following is the icon for the Favorites folder?

APPLY YOUR SKILLS

33. Create a new folder under C:\ and name it Transcription. Make this new folder the Default Working folder.

34. Open Explorer. Display the Status bar and the Address bar (if not already displayed). Display the file tree. Using the keyboard, move to the file list area. Change the view to Details. Sort by date.

35. Change your folder options to display hidden files and folders and display file extensions.

36. Locate the following files on your computer and write down the path name for each:

    Normal.dot   _____

    MSO1033.ACL   _____

    Custom.dic   _____

The Word Interface

INTRODUCTION

This lesson will introduce you to the many elements in the Word interface and how to control the way they appear. You will also learn about the many optional settings in MS Word. Understanding these settings is the key to making MS Word work efficiently for you.

Objectives:

1. Identify Elements in a Word window
2. Recognize document views
3. Identify main features and tools in Word
4. Adjust settings and options

READ AND WATCH

Chapter 4, pp 47–54 and Chapter 5, pp 55–80

Introduction to Word

TEST YOUR KNOWLEDGE

Answer the following questions:

1. List the four Mode buttons found on the Status bar and give the function of each.

_____

_____

2. List seven formatting properties indicated on the Horizontal ruler.

_____

_____

3. What can you do if a needed command on a menu is "grayed out" and therefore not available?

_____

_____

4. How do you access the dialogue box to change the way toolbars and menus behave?

_____

_____

5. What is a ScreenTip?

_____

_____

6. These formatting marks correspond to what key on the keyboard?

• _____

→ _____

¶ _____

7. Explain why formatting marks in Word are so important.

_____

_____

8. Explain the difference between boilerplates and templates as the terms are used in MS Word.

_____

_____

_____

9. Which Options box allows you to select different formatting marks (aka non-printing characters)?

_____

_____

10. Describe the recently-used file list.

_____

_____

11. Name two possible functions of the Insert key.

_____

_____

12. Which Options box shows you the path name for templates?

_____

_____

13. If the dictator requires words or phrases in uppercase, how can you make sure Word spellchecks these words?

_____

_____

14. Explain how you can turn off Automatic numbered lists.

_____

_____

15. Which three fractions will AutoFormat to a single-space fraction?

_____

_____

16. Explain how each of the following automatic features will affect your document if you have checked the boxes in the AutoFormat As You Type dialogue box.

Headings _____

_____

Borders _____

_____

Automatic numbered list _____

_____

17. Explain how to turn off the Office Assistant.

_____

_____

Fill in the blank:

Which tab under Tools>Options contains the following command?

18. Display field codes and shading   _____

19. Select which formatting marks to be displayed   _____

20. Recently-used file list   _____

21. Set user initials and default return address for envelopes   _____

22. Tabs and backspace set left indent   _____

23. AutoRecover settings   _____

24. Prompt to save Normal
    template   _____

25. Change grammar settings   _____

26. Check and recheck spelling   _____

Fill in the blank:

Where would you go to:

27. Disable the Task Pane on startup (in Word XP)

    _____

28. Disable Smart Tags (in Word XP)

    _____

29. Locate settings for Automatic Capitalization and TWo
    INitial CAps

    _____

30. Turn off AutoCorrect feature that automatically adds
    exceptions to the AutoCorrect list

    _____

31. Prevent Word from reformatting documents when opened
    on another computer

    _____

32. Prevent Word from re-defining a style when manual
    formatting is applied

    _____

Match these terms to their definitions:

Match these terms to the definition given below: AutoText,
AutoCorrect, Macro, Template, Boilerplate

33. _____ Layout of a given report.

34. _____ An actual file which Word uses for instructions on formatting, AutoText, macros, and customizations.

35. _____ A series of commands recorded as a single command.

36. _____ A built-in feature in Word that is used to store text and graphics.

37. _____ A built-in feature in Word that is used to automatically correct typos and misspelled words.

Identify these icons:

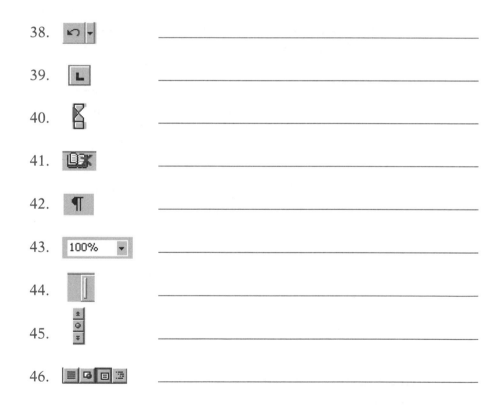

38. _____

39. _____

40. _____

41. _____

42. _____

43. _____

44. _____

45. _____

46. _____

Fill in the blank:

Which document view:

47. Shows text, graphics, headers and footers, and other elements as they will appear on the printed page. Displays the header and footer area and shows the entire page whether or not there is text.

_____

48. Shows only text formatting and no white space, page boundaries, headers, footers, backgrounds, drawing objects or pictures that do not have the In line with text wrapping style.

_____

49. Gives you a snapshot of what your document will look like when it actually prints on paper.

_____

Describe what happens:

Right-click on these objects:

50. Spelling and grammar icon   _____

51. TRK button   _____

52. Any toolbar   _____

Double-click these icons:

53. Blank spot to the right of the toolbars

_____

54. Page number on the Status bar

_____

55. REC on the Status bar   _____

56. TRK on the Status bar _____

57. EXT on the Status bar _____

58. OVR on the Status bar _____

59. Book icon _____

60. Gray space at either end of the Horizontal ruler

    _____

61. Lower gray bar of Horizontal ruler

    _____

62. Title bar _____

APPLY YOUR SKILLS

63. Step through the following:
    a. Open a document and change the view to Normal and then Print/Page Layout.
    b. Note the difference in each view.
    c. Which shows the most amount of information?
    d. Which shows the least amount of information?
    e. View the document in Full Screen Mode.
    f. View the document with paragraph marks on and off.

64. Open Tools>Options>Edit. Right-click each option and read its description.

65. Open Tools>Options>View. Right-click each of these options and read the description: Status bar, Screen tips, Horizontal scroll bar, Vertical scroll bar, and All (under formatting marks).

66. Step through the following:

  a. Open Tools>Options>General.

  b. Set the Recently used file list to 9.

  c. Close the dialogue box.

  d. Open three different Word documents.

  e. Use the File menu and the Recently used file list to switch between these three files.

  f. Close the files and use the keyboard and the Recently used file list to open one of the files.

67. Open Tools>Options>Save. Check AutoRecover info and change to every 3 minutes.

68. Open Tools>Options>Grammar. Remove the check mark at Ignore words in Uppercase.

69. Go to Tools>AutoCorrect.

  a. Remove the check mark at Automatically use suggestions from the spelling checker.

  b. Remove check marks at Exceptions>Automatically add words to list (all three tabs).

  c. Right-click the command to automatically add words to list and read the explanation.

70. Go to Tools>Templates and Add-ins. Remove the check mark at Automatically update document styles.

Formatting

INTRODUCTION

Formatting fonts and paragraphs is the most fundamental task in a word processor. This lesson will explain how Word applies formatting, how to interpret formatting information, and also how to format the most common special characters and paragraph types used in medical transcription.

Objectives:

1. Define formatting marks
2. Understand the role of the insertion point
3. Apply formatting commands
4. Interpret formatting information in a graphical interface
5. Set defaults
6. Format common paragraph types used in transcription
7. Troubleshoot formatting problems
8. Format headers and footers
9. Manage automatically numbered lists
10. Use tables

READ AND WATCH

Chapter 7, pp 91–115 and Chapter 13, pp 161–172

Format a SOAP note

TEST YOUR KNOWLEDGE

Answer the following questions:

1. Define "Interactive Interface."

   _____

   _____

2. Toolbars and rulers display formatting information based on the location of what element on the screen?

   _____

   _____

3. What happens every time you press the Enter key?

   _____

   _____

4. List two ways to apply formatting to a word.

   _____

   _____

5. How do you change the Default font?

   _____

   _____

6. Give the shortcut keys for superscript and subscript formatting.

   _____

   _____

7. Explain a nonbreaking space and a nonbreaking hyphen.

   _____

   _____

8. Define a paragraph in MS Word.

_____

_____

9. New paragraphs have what formatting?

_____

_____

10. Explain these characteristics of paragraph formatting.

Alignment _____

_____

Indentation _____

_____

11. Explain two ways to define (i.e., set) tab stops.

_____

_____

_____

12. How do you determine the depth of indents and hanging indents?

_____

_____

13. Describe hanging indent.

_____

_____

14. Give the shortcut key for formatting a paragraph as a hanging indent.

_____

15. A SOAP note uses which two paragraph types?

_____

_____

16. Give the shortcut keys for aligning paragraphs.

Left   _____

Right   _____

Center   _____

Justified _____

17. Give the shortcut key for displaying font and paragraph
formatting information (i.e., Reveal codes or "What's this?")

_____

18. Give the shortcut key for removing manual paragraph
formatting.

_____

19. How do you access the dialogue box to set page margins?

_____

_____

20. List two reasons for inserting a section break.

_____

_____

21. How do you insert a section break?

_____

_____

22. Which view does not display headers and footers?

_____

_____

23. How do you make the first page header look different than the second and subsequent pages?

_____

_____

24. In order to have different headers in each section, what command must be changed?

_____

_____

25. How do you end an automatically numbered list?

_____

_____

26. What is the shortcut key for moving an indented list back to the left margin in Word 2000 and XP (when Automatic numbering is turned on)?

_____

27. Explain the difference between the Automatic numbered list feature and the Numbered list format.

_____

_____

_____

28. Describe two ways to create a list within a list (sub list) when Automatic numbering is turned on.

_____

_____

_____

29. Explain how to repair an automatically numbered list when the numbering or format within the list is incorrect.

_____

_____

30. If an automatically numbered list starts with the wrong number (i.e., not number 1), how do you correct the numbering?

_____

_____

31. Describe how you would delete a table's contents as opposed to deleting the table itself.

_____

_____

_____

32. How can you convert text to a table format?

_____

_____

33. How do you insert a tab in a table cell?

_____

_____

Match-up the following icons:

Match these icons to its corresponding command.

34. ▣   Toggle Header and Footer link

35. ▣   Page Setup dialogue box

36. ▣   Page number field

37. ▣   Date field

38. ▣   Total number of pages field

Interpret:

39. List the formatting commands applied to the paragraph represented by these toolbars:

_____

_____

_____

APPLY YOUR SKILLS

Using the keyboard and shortcut keys, format the following terms with subscripts and superscripts:

40. H_2O, CO_2, hemoglobin A_{1c}, FEV_1, Lead aV_R, Lead aV_F

41. ^{123}I, ^{131}I, cm^2, mm^3

Insert these symbols into a document:

42. α (alpha)

43. β (beta)

44. ° (degree symbol)

Type the following paragraphs using nonbreaking spaces between titles and surnames and also within the medication dose to keep dose and form together (i.e., 30 mg). Use a nonbreaking hyphen between the hyphenated surnames.

45. Dr. Smith ordered the following medications for Mrs. Jones-Harvey: Prevacid 30 mg, ibuprofen 200 mg. Mr. Harvey will help Mrs. Jones-Harvey return to the clinic next week for a followup appointment.

46. The patient is scheduled to see her new psychiatrist Dr. Jones-Smith who will refer her to the neurologist Dr. James-Henry. I will change her antidepressant medication today from Prozac 20 mg twice a day to Zoloft 100 mg.

Turn on Automatic numbered lists (Tools>AutoCorrect>AutoFormat As You Type). Type the following numbered list and insert a sublist as shown below:

47.

1. Cardiovascular disease.

    a. Status post myocardial infarction.

    b. Status post congestive heart failure.

2. Hypertension.

3. Diabetes mellitus.

48.

1. Pulmonary hypertension.

    a. Status post congestive heart failure.

    b. Status post pneumonia.

2. Diabetes mellitus.

3. Obesity.

49. Turn off Automatic numbered lists (Tools>AutoCorrect> AutoFormat As You Type) and format the following using shortcut keys to format the indents and hanging indents:

Axis I: 1. Adjustment disorder with mixed anxiety and depressed mood (309.28), chronic.
2. Psychosocial factors having an adverse affect on ability to respond to medical treatment.

Axis II: No Diagnosis

Axis III: Obtained from medical record:

1. Lumbar radiculopathy, chronic, status post lumbar interbody fusion at L4–L5.
2. Lumbar facet syndrome, chronic, status post steroid injections X2.

Axis IV: No diagnosis.

Axis V: Current GAF = 60. Highest GAF in the Past Year = 65.

50. Format the following SOAP note using indent and hanging indent commands. Do not use the tab key to indent text.

S: The patient returns today for further evaluation of fatigue, nausea, vomiting and general malaise. Since her last visit, she has improved only slightly with the use of Phenergan.

O: Today she is in no acute distress. Blood pressure is 130/80, pulse 80, respirations 16, temperature 99.0°. No abdominal masses. Right upper quadrant tenderness unchanged since last visit.

A: 1. Gastroenteritis following recent travel outside the country. Suspect viral etiology.
2. Peptic ulcer disease.
3. Hypertension, controlled on current medication.

P: 1. Continue to push fluids with strict bed rest. RICE diet for 3 days and then advance as tolerated.
2. Phenergan p.r.n.
3. Return to clinic in 1 week.

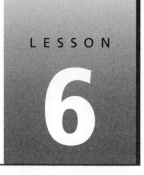
Templates and Fields

INTRODUCTION

This lesson will introduce template files in MS Word. These files are invaluable for creating consistent documents quickly and easily. Template files contain more than just standard text; they contain all the elements needed to create a document including formatting, margins, and customizations. In addition to setting up template files, you will also learn how to automate documents using fields and how to set markers or "jump" points for navigating through a document using blank fields.

Objectives:

1. Understand the role of Normal.dot and template files
2. Create and use document templates
3. Modify a document template
4. Use the Organizer to manage templates
5. Use empty fields as markers
6. Use common fields

READ AND WATCH

Chapter 8, pp 117–127 and Chapter 11, pp. 147–152

Create a New Template File
Using the Organizer

TEST YOUR KNOWLEDGE

Answer the following questions:

1. Define a template file.

   _____

   _____

2. Which template file is always active?

   _____

   _____

3. Name eight elements of a template file.

   _____

   _____

4. What is the difference between a global template and a document template?

   _____

   _____

5. Unless you specify otherwise, shortcuts, macros, and customizations are stored in which template?

   _____

   _____

6. Why is it important to back up the Normal.dot?

   _____

   _____

7. How do you designate a file as a template?

   _____

   _____

8. How do you open a new document *based* on a template?

    _____

9. How do you modify a template file?

    _____

    _____

10. Describe the Organizer dialogue box.

    _____

    _____

    _____

11. Explain "File in use by another user?"

    _____

    _____

12. What is the shortcut key to insert an empty field?

    _____

    _____

13. What is the shortcut key to jump to an empty field?

    _____

    _____

14. If your Page up and Page down keys change function, how can you fix this?

    _____

    _____

15. How do you format an empty field?

    _____

    _____

16. How can you use an empty field to give notes and instructions?

    _____

    _____

17. Name three types of fields that might be useful in transcription.

    _____

    _____

18. Which type of date field would be better to use for medical transcription and why?

    _____

    _____

19. What shortcut key will hide or display field codes?

    _____

    _____

APPLY YOUR SKILLS

Follow these steps to set up a template file:

20. Open a new document and save the document as a template (dot file). Name it Sample.dot.

21. Set the default page margins at 1 inch top and bottom and 1.25 inches left and right. Set the default font as Times New Roman 12 point.

22. Type the headings and the standard text as shown in the document labeled "Office Consultation" on page 222 of the *Guide*. Format the past medical history section using tables as shown.

23. Insert blank fields where shown in the template. Set font formatting so that the name inserts in bold and uppercase. Leave a note to the transcriptionist to type allergies in bold if the standard phrase "No known drug allergies" is replaced.

24. Insert a page break if necessary to create a second page.

25. Open the Page Setup dialogue box and switch to the Layout tab. Place a check mark at Different first page.

26. Open the header space and place headings for the patient name, date of service, and page number on the second page.

27. In the header space, insert a field for the page number.

28. Delete the page break.

29. Save the changes and close the template file.

30. Create a document based on the template file you just created and name it Consultation.doc.

31. Repeat steps 20–30 above to create a new template. Format the document using the sample on page 220 of the *Guide* as an example.

Increasing Productivity with AutoText, AutoCorrect and Macros

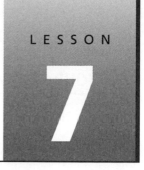

LESSON

7

INTRODUCTION

This lesson will focus on three features built into MS Word that the transcriptionist can use to increase production while maintaining quality. Choosing the correct "tool" for the job is important, so this lesson will give specific examples of how to apply these features and also explain how to troubleshoot common problems.

Objectives:

1. Use AutoCorrect
2. Use AutoText
3. Use the Macro Recorder
4. Backup, copy, and restore productivity data
5. Troubleshoot common problems in AutoText and AutoCorrect
6. Identify key differences between AutoText, AutoCorrect, and Macros

READ AND WATCH

Chapter 9, pp 129–138, Chapter 10, pp 139–146, and Chapter 12, pp 153–160

Create a Formatted AutoCorrect Entry
Record a Macro
Correct Capitalization Macro

TEST YOUR KNOWLEDGE

Answer the following questions:

1. What is the intended use of AutoCorrect?

   _____

   _____

2. List at least four ways to use AutoCorrect.

   _____

   _____

3. How do you access the AutoCorrect dialogue box?

   _____

   _____

4. Why must you be very careful when designating a shortcut for an AutoCorrect entry?

   _____

   _____

5. How do you create an AutoCorrect entry?

   _____

   _____

6. How do you create an AutoCorrect entry with formatting?

   _____

   _____

7. How do you insert an AutoCorrect entry?

   _____

   _____

8. Explain how to create an AutoCorrect entry during a
    spell check.

    _____

    _____

9. What shortcut key will reverse an AutoCorrect correction?

    _____

    _____

10. What two files are necessary to completely back up your
    AutoCorrect entries?

    _____

    _____

11. Compare and contrast AutoCorrect and AutoText.

    _____

    _____

    _____

12. List two ways to memorize an AutoText entry.

    _____

    _____

13. List two ways to insert an AutoText entry.

    _____

    _____

    _____

14. Explain how to designate a template to store AutoText entries.

_____

_____

_____

15. Why is it important to designate the Default font when using AutoText?

_____

_____

_____

16. Which dialogue box will let you easily copy AutoText entries to another template?

_____

_____

17. Name two ways to delete an AutoText entry.

_____

_____

18. Describe the best application of a Macro in MS Word.

_____

_____

19. List at least two specific ways you could use a Macro in Word.

_____

_____

20. List two ways of accessing the Record Macro dialogue box.

_____

_____

21. Give the rules for naming a Macro.

_____

_____

22. How do you back up Macros?

_____

_____

Match-up:

What method would be the best choice for the following shortcuts: AutoText (AT), AutoCorrect (AC), Macros (M), or templates (.dot file)? Briefly explain why.

23. Change qd to q.d. _____

24. Format cc: so that the first c is not capped _____

25. CO_2 _____

26. Dr. with a nonbreaking space included in the shortcut _____

27. "eat" as a shortcut for "evaluation and treatment" _____

28. Thirty SOAP formats, one right after the other _____

29. A standard diabetic review of systems used in about 20% of reports _____

30. Change a comma to a period and capitalize the next word

_____

31. Delete a "risk and benefit" disclaimer from an H&P when not needed _____

32. A physical exam paragraph_____

33. Correct a common typo such as hedaache_____

34. Create a shortcut containing a field_____

35. A database of 500 addresses_____

36. A letterhead with specific fonts, different than the font in the body of the letter_____

APPLY YOUR SKILLS

Create AutoCorrect entries for the following:

37. t.i.d.

38. q.i.d.

39. change cbc to CBC

40. H_2O

41. CO_2

42. lead aV_R

43. ^{123}I

44. -year-old

Create AutoText entries for:

45. cc: (including the tab space)

46. The SOAP note format created in Lesson 6

47. Main headings shown in the sample template on page 219 of the *Guide*

48. Create a template file and use the AutoText headings created in #47 above to insert the headings into your new template file.

Record these macros:

49. Open a new document based on a template as described on page 225 of the *Guide*.

50. Correct missed caps after a colon described on page 232 of the *Guide*.

Editing

INTRODUCTION

Proofing and editing documents can be time-consuming, yet important for creating accurate medical records. This lesson will show you how to edit more efficiently using several different techniques and also how to manage the spelling and grammar checking functions. In addition, shortcut keys will be covered in more depth. The last part of the lesson will cover electronic research techniques.

Objectives:

1. Use shortcut keys to move around in a document
2. Use the Spelling and Grammar checker
3. Edit the Custom dictionary
4. Adjust Grammar and Language
5. Edit text using shortcut keys
6. Use Word tools: Find, Replace, Copy, Extend, Spike
7. Research information using electronic references

READ AND WATCH

 Chapter 6, pp. 81–90 and Chapter 14, pp. 173–193.

 Edit the Custom Dictionary
Print a list of Shortcut Keys

TEST YOUR KNOWLEDGE

Answer the following questions:

1. List at least three ways to spell check a document.

    _____

    _____

2. Explain these two icons: 🔲 and 🔲

    _____

    _____

3. What is the function of the Add command on the Spelling and Grammar dialogue box and shortcut menu?

    _____

    _____

4. Explain the difference between the Main dictionary and the Custom dictionary.

    _____

    _____

    _____

5. Describe two ways to remove a word from the Custom dictionary.

    _____

    _____

6. In Word 97 or Word 2000, what must you do after editing the Custom dictionary?

    _____

    _____

7. Describe at least two ways to obtain formatting
    information from Word.

    _____

    _____

8. How can you print a list of shortcut keys assigned to macros?

    _____

    _____

9. What happens when you press the shift key along with
    the arrow keys?

    _____

    _____

10. Give the position of the cursor (insertion point) after
    pressing the following keys:

    Home   _____

    End   _____

    CTL+Home   _____

    CTL+End   _____

11. List three ways to close a document using the keyboard.

    _____

    _____

12. Give the shortcut key for "repeat the last action?"

    _____

    _____

13. List the shortcut key for placing the insertion point at the
    previous revision (edit).

    _____

    _____

14. Give the shortcut keys for:

Bold   _____

Italic   _____

Underline   _____

Redo last action   _____

Change case of letters   _____

Open the Save As dialog box _____

Open the Font dialog box   _____

15. Explain the use of the F8 key.

_____

_____

_____

16. Name four separate uses of the Undo command.

_____

_____

17. Explain how you would locate and delete (in one step) a
word used several times in a document.

_____

_____

Match-up:

Match the commands with these shortcut keys:

18.	CTRL+Q	Format selected text as all caps
19.	CTRL+Spacebar	Decrease the font size by 1 point
20.	CTRL+F	Copy the formatting commands for the selected text
21.	CTRL+H	Remove manual formatting from a paragraph
22.	CTRL+G	Insert a manual page break
23.	CTRL+F2	Apply copied formatting commands to the selected text
24.	CTRL+[	Remove manual formatting from text
25.	CTRL+Shift+A	Move to the beginning of the previous paragraph
26.	CTRL+Shift+C	Delete one word to the left
27.	CTRL+Shift+V	Open the Find dialogue box
28.	CTRL+Backspace	Open the Go To dialogue box
29.	CTRL+Enter	Change the View to Print Preview
30.	CTRL+Up arrow	Open the Find and Replace dialogue box

Give an explanation:

31. What happens when the Arrow key is pressed when text is selected?

   _____

   _____

32. Explain how the Shift key affects the navigation keys.

   _____

   _____

33. Explain how to adjust the grammar settings in MS Word.

   _____

   _____

   _____

APPLY YOUR SKILLS

34. Add an incorrect word to the Custom dictionary. Remove the word from the list by editing the Custom dictionary.

35. Use the "What's This?" command and click on text that contains formatting such as those created in the lesson on formatting. Write down the formatting information displayed.

   Formatting defined by the style:

   _____

   _____

   Formatting added on top of a style:

   _____

   _____

36. Use the Extend mode to delete a word.

37. Use the Extend mode to delete a sentence.

38. Use the Extend mode to delete the last half of a sentence.

39. Use the Extend mode along with the Find feature to select text from the beginning of the document to a particular word used within the document. (Press F8, CTRL+F, type the word, press Enter, press Esc)

40. Print the list of Word commands using the ListCommands macro.

Customizing Word

INTRODUCTION

Word is quite flexible and can be changed in many ways to suit the user's needs. Customizing Word can significantly increase your productivity. This lesson will show you the many ways Word can be customized, including menus, toolbars, and shortcut key assignments.

Objectives:

1. Customize toolbars
2. Customize menus
3. Customize shortcut keys

READ AND WATCH

Chapter 15, pp. 195–205

Customize Menus in Word
Customize Toolbars in Word
Create a Work Menu

TEST YOUR KNOWLEDGE

Answer the following questions:

1. List the different features in Word that can be customized.

_____

_____

2. List three ways to open the Customize dialogue box.

_____

_____

3. What must be showing in order to access the drop-down menu to customize a button on a toolbar?

_____

_____

4. Where can you find a list of over 400 commands that can be added to menus and toolbars?

_____

_____

5. Describe a simple method of moving an icon to a new location on a toolbar.

_____

_____

6. Describe a simple method of copying an existing icon from one toolbar to another toolbar.

_____

_____

7. When customizing a toolbar or menu command, what symbol is used to assign a hot key?

_____

_____

8. How do you access the Customize Keyboard dialogue box?

_____

_____

9.   Describe two ways to use the ALT key.

_____

_____

10.   Shortcut keys must contain at least one of these keys:

_____

_____

11.   Which tab on the Customize dialogue box is used to create a new toolbar?

_____

_____

12.   Which tab of the Customize dialogue box is used to create a new menu?

_____

_____

APPLY YOUR SKILLS

Assign shortcut keys to these commands:

13.   SentLeft

14.   SentRight

15.   TableDeleteRow

16.   TableDeleteColumn

17.   ToolsAutoCorrect (to open the AutoCorrect dialogue box)

Complete these projects:

18.   Complete the project described on page 224 of the _Guide_ to create a new toolbar.

19.   Complete the project on page 225 of the _Guide_ to create a Work menu.

20.   Add a new command or macro to the Text/Text shortcut menu.

Problem Solving

Below are a list of typical problems encountered by transcriptionists using MS Word. Test your knowledge and see if you know the solution to the problem.

1. You notice that you misspelled "PENICILLIN" (typed in all caps), but Word did not mark it with a red wavy line. What should you do?

2. Suddenly you have red and blue lines in your document (underscores and strikeouts). What should you do?

3. After inserting the AutoText entry "The patient returns for followup," the insertion point moves to the next line. What should you do?

4. After creating an AutoText entry for "The patient comes in today," you do not get a suggestion box. What should you do?

5. You notice there are words that are not capitalized even though they start a sentence. What should you do?

6. You created several macros that would be helpful to other MTs who work on the same account. How could you share these macros with them?

7. You created a template that has the office letterhead in the header space on the first page but you want to put patient information on the second page. What should you do?

8. You just finished typing a document and the patient's diagnosis was Ménière's disease. Now, spell check is suggesting words in French. What should you do?

9. You are using a work station that belonged to another MT and you have found several incorrect words that appear on the suggestion list during a spell check. What should you do?

10. When typing a numbered list, it always indents. What do you do if you need it to line up at the left margin?

11. You created a shortcut in AutoCorrect for "b.i.d." but you need to type the word "bid." What is the easiest way to solve this problem?

12. During a tech support call, the technician asks you what version of Windows you are running and what type of processor is installed. How do you find the answers?

13. The office calls and asks you to email a copy of a file that you transcribed about two weeks ago. The only information they can give you is the patient's last name. What do you do?

14. You need to devise a way to quickly access a group of folders and their files. Explain how you might do this (you can use the mouse to set up the system, but you want to use the keyboard to use the system).

15. You have a list of 20 Internet sites that you use on a regular basis. How would you set up shortcuts for these so you can access them using the keyboard?

16. You need to locate and delete about 20 files that have the name "jones" included in the file name. This folder contains over 200 files. What is the easiest way to do this?

17. You are running Windows XP, but you prefer the way the Start menu and the folders appeared in Windows 98. What can you do?

18. You have created a template that includes several standard paragraphs. About 20% of the time, the dictator asks you to delete the standard and replace it with a different standard. How can you do this with a single keystroke?

19. You have the opportunity to take a trip but you must continue to work. A friend has offered to loan you her laptop. What can you do to make your shortcuts available?

20. You are working in a document and suddenly every time you strike another key, more text is selected. What has happened?

21. You created a new document yesterday, but you do not remember the file name or the folder. How can you find this file?

22. You were given a sample document for a new account. You have used this file to create new files, but at least once a day you forget to rename the file, so the original is changed. What would be the best solution?

23. You have been working on a particularly difficult dictation during a thunderstorm. If you MUST continue working in spite of an impending storm, what can you do to safeguard your work?

24. You accidentally pasted a large amount of text into the middle of a document. What is the easiest way to fix this?

25. You have been asked to proof some documents typed by a new transcriptionist. You notice there is a misspelled word that is not marked. What should you do to check for other possible spelling errors?

26. Word always abbreviates the drop-down menus, making you click at the bottom of the menu to see the entire list of menu choices. What can you do to change this behavior?

27. How would you set formatting in all caps and bold as part of the template so that the transcriptionist does not have to apply formatting while typing?

28. You have set up a series of template files (dot files) that you use regularly. You need to be able to modify these templates fairly often. What can you do to easily access these templates?

Answer Key

LESSON ONE

1. Keys written with a plus sign should be pressed together, while keys written with a comma are pressed sequentially.

2. They are marked by an underscore (line).

3. The first character of an object's name

4. A list of commands grouped by specific types of tasks

5. Press the ALT key, followed by the underscored letter.

6. Indicates the active window, gives the name of the application and the current file, and contains the window-control commands: maximize, minimize, restore, size, and close commands.

7. Press the ALT key to activate the Title bar, press the Spacebar to open the Control menu, and then press the letter 'n.'

8. The Logo key

9. Logo+E

10. Logo+D or Logo+M

11. To manage applications, folders, or windows that are currently open

12. The Home key (to the beginning) and the End key (to the end)

13. The Copy command places text, graphics or other objects on the clipboard to be pasted to a new location. The Paste command inserts the object that is currently stored on the clipboard. The Cut command copies the selected object to the clipboard and removes it from the original location.

14. CTRL+A

15. F2

16. Backspace

17. The + sign indicates that the folder contains subfolders. The − sign indicates that the folder is expanded and subfolders are displayed.

18. Tap the alpha character, i.e., the first letter of the drive or folder name. Repeat the letter if there is more than one folder with the same initial character.

19. A separate window within an application that allows you to change settings and options

20. Press the Tab key to move from one command to the next or press ALT+hot key to jump directly to a command.

21. Use ALT+hot key or press CTL+Tab.

22. The Spacebar

23. By a dotted line around the command or button name or by highlighting a command in a drop-down box

24. Press the Esc key.

25. Close the current window or the application.

26. Switch to another open window.

27. Copy

28. Paste

29. Cut

30. Open the Search pane.

31. Help

32. Open the Address bar.

33. Close a dialogue box or cancel an action.

34. Toggle to a different pane in the same window.

35. Open Windows Search (Find).

36. Activate the Menu bar.

37. Open System Properties dialogue box.

38. Open the Close Program dialogue box or the Security dialogue box in Windows XP.

39. H:\Laura\Pulm

40. Detail view

LESSON TWO

1. A right-click menu which changes commands depending on the object clicked.

2. An object can be a file, folder, shortcut icon, application icon, toolbar, graphic, word, or a selection of text and/or graphics.

3. Behavior and settings

4. Right-click on the Desktop away from any other object and choose Properties.

5. Right-click on a blank area of the Taskbar and choose Tile Windows Horizontally.

6. Right-click on the option or command and choose "What's This?"

7. Open, Edit, Print, Cut, Copy, Create Shortcut, Delete, Rename, Properties, Send to

8. Copy a file to another drive or folder, email a file, create a shortcut on the Desktop, or compress a file.

9. You actually send a copy of the shortcut to the email recipient, not the actual file.

10. Files are copied if the original location and the send-to location are on different drives. The file is moved if the two locations are on the same drive.

11. The Application key

12. Shortcuts have a small curved arrow in the bottom left corner of the icon.

13. No, shortcuts do not move the actual file.

14. No, the shortcut can have any name.

15. There is no limit to the number of shortcuts that can be placed on the Start menu.

16. Point to an object with the mouse cursor, hold down the left mouse button and drag the object toward another object. Continue holding the mouse button and hover the pointer over the target object and release the mouse button.

17. Hold down the modifier key on the keyboard while clicking an object with the mouse button. CTRL+Click allows you to choose items in a list that are not contiguous. Shift+Click allows you to select a range of items in a list.

18. Hold down the modifier key on the keyboard while dragging the object with the left mouse button.

19. Normal select

20. "What's this?" or Help mode

21. Precision select

22. Resize mode

23. Move mode

24. Go to Link

LESSON THREE

1. A three-character identifier that follows the last period in a file name. Windows (the operating system) uses this extension to identify the type of file and the application associated with the file.

2. .doc (Word), .xls (Excel), .txt (text file), .exe (an executable file, typically used to launch a program.)

3. Also called a directory, a folder contains related files and possibly more folders. Windows uses folders to locate files much like the post office uses your address to locate your house.

4. Windows does not set a limit to the number of folders you can create.

5. Information Windows uses to run your computer and the different applications you have installed

6. The unique address or location of a file. The path name includes the drive, folder, and any subfolders containing the file.

7. A single backslash indicates the file is located on the computer you are working on. The two forward slashes mean the file is located on another computer connected to yours by a network (including web sites).

8. A utility in Windows for managing the files and folders on your computer

9. Yes

10. Rename, delete, copy, view properties, move files, create new folders, open, and save files

11. My Documents (the Default working folder)

12. Press Shift+Tab.

13. Click the View icon and choose Arrange icons OR change the view to Details and then click the column header to sort by that header.

14. List, Details, Icon, Tiles, Thumbnails

15. Shortcuts to files, folders, drives, and Internet sites

16. Moving from folder to folder or moving from one web site to another

17. Change the setting in Windows to display Hidden files and folders. This command is found on the Tools menu under Folder options on the View tab. In Windows 98, the option is found under the View menu.

18. You can use any piece of known information such as the file type, the file extension, the file name or a part of the file name, a word contained within the file, a date range when the file was last modified, or the file size.

19. * (asterisk) substitutes for any number of unknown characters; ? (question mark) means any one character

20. Right-click and choose commands such as Open, Print, Send to (email, create shortcut), Copy, Cut, Delete, Rename, view Properties.

21. Normal.dot, AutoCorrect file, Custom dictionary

22. Press CTRL+S periodically.

23. AutoRecover must be turned on and the file must be named.

24. Open Word. Recovered documents will automatically be opened. Use the Save As command to rename the recovered file back to the original file name in the original file location (folder).

25. Open the Close Program dialogue box (or Task Manager if using XP). If Winword appears on the list, select and click the End Task command. Re-open the dialogue box to make sure Winword no longer appears on the list. Now, re-open Word and recover your documents if necessary.

26. Return to previous folder.

27. Go up one folder level.

28. Open Internet Explorer.

29. Delete the selected item.

30. Create a new folder.

31. Open Views.

32. The icon with the starbust in the center of the folder. The icon with the starburst in the corner of the folder is the New folder icon.

LESSON FOUR

1. REC turns on the Macro recorder (Record mode).

   TRK turns on Track Changes (also called Revision marks).

   EXT turns on Extend mode for selecting text.

   OVR turns on Overtype mode for deleting text as you type instead of inserting text.

2. Left and right page margins, tab type and tab location, paragraph indention, first-line indent, right indent, hanging indent

3. Move the insertion point or select some text or an object on the page that relates to the command needed.

4. Tools>Customize>Options tab OR right-click anywhere within the toolbar area and choose Customize.

5. A brief description that appears when you hover the mouse pointer over an icon

6. ● Spacebar

   → Tab key

   ¶ Enter key

7. Formatting marks actually store formatting information. The paragraph mark carries a hard return plus any formatting information for the preceding paragraph. Tabs and spaces also carry font formatting.

8. A boilerplate is standard text. Typically, the boilerplate has the layout of any one particular report type, including the headings and the patient demographic information and signature line. A template, on the other hand, is an actual file. It can contain boilerplate text, but it also contains formatting information such as page layout, fonts, key assignments, customized menus, toolbars and shortcut keys, macros, and styles.

9. Tools>Options>View

10. A list of the most recently opened/used files which appears at the bottom of the File menu in Word and many other programs. This list can be used to quickly open the files it contains.

11. It can be used to enable Overtype mode or it can be used as the Paste command.

12. Tools>Options>File Locations

13. Go to Tools>Options>Spelling and Grammar tab and remove the check mark at Ignore words in uppercase.

14. Tools>AutoCorrect>AutoFormat As You Type, clear the check mark at Automatic numbered lists

15. $\frac{1}{4}$, $\frac{1}{2}$, and $\frac{3}{4}$

16. Headings: Word will "assume" centered and bold text is a heading and will apply a heading style, or Word will create a new heading style. If a paragraph following a heading style has manual formatting applied, Word will create a new body text style.

    Borders: Word will change three or more underscored characters into a border (a line extending the width of the page).

Automatic numbered lists: Word will "detect" a list when you type a number followed by a tab and then text. When you press the Enter key, Word will insert the next number in the list and format the list with a hanging indent.

17. Right-click on the Assistant, choose Options. Remove the check mark at Use the Office Assistant.

18. View

19. View

20. General

21. User Information

22. Edit or Tools>AutoCorrect>AutoFormat As you Type in Word XP

23. Save

24. Save

25. Spelling and Grammar

26. Spelling and Grammar

27. Tools>Options>View

28. Tools>Options>View

29. Tools>AutoCorrect

30. Tools>AutoCorrect>Exceptions (all three tabs)

31. Tools>Templates and Add-ins

32. Tools>AutoCorrect>AutoFormat As You Type

33. Boilerplate

34. Template

35. Macro

36. AutoText

37. AutoCorrect

38. Undo

39. Tab type indicator, left-aligned tab

40. Indent commands on the Horizontal ruler

41. Spelling and Grammar icon

42. Show/Hide formatting marks

43. Zoom

44. Toolbar handle

45. Browse by

46. Page view buttons

47. Print/Page Layout

48. Normal

49. Print Preview

50. A menu appears with spelling and grammar commands

51. Opens a menu to adjust Track changes

52. Opens a menu to hide or display toolbars

53. Opens the Customize dialogue box

54. Opens the Go To dialogue box

55. Opens the Record Macro dialogue box

56. Starts Track changes

57. Turns on Extend mode

58. Turns on Overtype mode

59. Selects the next misspelled word and opens the shortcut menu

60. Opens the Page Setup dialogue box to the Margins tab

61. Opens the Tab dialogue box

62. Maximizes or Restores window

LESSON FIVE

1. The icons on the screen are used for giving and receiving information (i.e., commands). The icons appear differently when the command is active.

2. The insertion point

3. A new paragraph is created every time you strike the Enter key.

4. Turn on the formatting before typing the word, type the word, then turn the formatting off OR place the insertion point anywhere within the word and then apply the formatting command.

5. Either change the definition of the Normal style OR use the Font dialogue box. Press CTRL+D to open the Font dialogue box, make the appropriate font changes and then click Default in the lower left corner. Answer Yes in the confirmation box.

6. Subscript is CTL+= (equal) and Superscript is CTL+Shift+= (equal).

7. A nonbreaking space prevents two words from separating across a line break. The two words are treated as if they are a single word, but the space remains for readability. The nonbreaking hyphen inserts a hyphen between two words but does not allow the words to separate across a line break.

8. Any text (or no text) that immediately precedes a paragraph mark. A blank line, a single word, several words or sentences or a centered heading are all considered paragraphs.

9. The same formatting as the paragraph above it, unless the preceding paragraph contains a command as part of the style to change the following paragraph (for example, heading styles are usually followed by a body text style).

10. Alignment refers to the horizontal placement of text relative to the margins. Paragraphs can be aligned even with the left margin, even with the right margin, justified so that they are even with both margins or centered between the margins.

    Indentation refers to the distance of the text from the page margin. The first line of a paragraph can have a different indentation than the rest of the paragraph.

11. Set the insertion point in the paragraph that will contain the tabs. Click the Tab Type indicator button to set the type of tab and then click the tab position on the Horizontal ruler. Or, you can open the Tab dialogue box (under the Format menu) and type in a tab location and check the button to indicate the tab type (right- or left-aligned, centered, etc). Click Set before closing the dialogue box.

12. By defining tab stops

13. The first line of a paragraph is closer to the left margin than the subsequent lines of the paragraph. This is the paragraph style most often used in numbered lists.

14. CTRL+T

15. Indent and Hanging indent

16. Left CTRL+L

    Right CTRL+R

    Center CTRL+E

    Justified CTRL+J

17. Shift+F1

18. CTRL+Q

19. File menu, Page setup dialogue box, Margins tab.

20. To change the headers and footers within a single document or to change the page margins within a document.

21. Open the Insert menu, choose Break. In the dialogue box, choose the type of section break needed.

22. Normal view

23. In the Page Setup dialogue box, on the Layout tab, place a check mark at Different first page.

24. Remove the command "Same as previous" from each section of the document.

25. Press the Enter key twice OR Backspace to delete the last number.

26. ALT+Shift+Left arrow

27. The automatic numbered list feature instructs Word to detect the start of a numbered list and automatically apply the numbered list format (insert list numbers and apply list format paragraph commands). The numbered list format is a style that defines a list as a hanging indent with numbers added to each list item. The format can be applied at any time to a list of items.

28. Use the Line break command to start a new line without starting a new list number, or select the text to be part of the sub list and apply the Demote command (ALT+Shift+Right arrow). A third method is to use the SkipNumbering command.

29. Select the entire list, click the Automatic numbering icon (on the Formatting toolbar) twice.

30. Place the insertion point in the first list item (i.e., the first paragraph). Right-click and choose Bullets and Numbering or choose Bullets and Numbering from the Format menu. Apply the command in the lower left corner "Restart numbering."

31. To delete just the text but not the table, select the cells (columns and rows) within the table and press the Delete key. To delete the table, place the insertion point anywhere within the table and choose Table>Delete>Table or use the shortcut keys ALT+Shift+5 to select the table and then press Delete.

32. Select the text, go to Table>Convert>Text to table. Choose the number of columns and indicate the character to be used to separate the text into columns.

33. CTRL+Tab

34. Date field

35. Page number field

36. Total number of pages field

37. Page Setup dialogue box

38. Toggle Header and Footer link (Same as previous command)

39. Formatting marks are displayed, the Zoom is set to 130%. The text is in the Normal style, Times New Roman 11 pt. with italic and subscript applied. The paragraph is left-aligned with automatic numbering applied. A tab is defined at 1.5 inches, the paragraph is indented to the 1-inch mark, and the hanging indent is set to the 1.5-inch mark. Page margins are set to 0.5 inches on the right and the left.

LESSON SIX

1. A file that contains settings such as font, margins, styles, custom toolbars and menus, macros, and standard text

2. The Normal.dot

3. Page Setup, Standard text, AutoText, Fonts and Styles, Toolbars, Menus, Key assignments, Macros

4. Global templates contain settings that apply to all documents. The Normal.dot is a global template. Document templates only apply to documents created using that template.

5. The Normal.dot

6. Because it is integral to running MS Word and it often becomes corrupt. It also contains important information and shortcuts such as AutoCorrect and AutoText entries and macros.

7. By saving it with the extension .dot

8. Open the File menu and choose the New command. Choose the template from the New dialogue box. In XP, the New document task pane will open. Choose General templates and choose the template name from the dialogue box.

9. Click the Open command, navigate to the template folder, choose the template and click Open. You cannot open it using the File>New dialogue box.

10. The Organizer allows the user to copy AutoText, Macros, Styles and Toolbars between two different template files. It contains two panes, one to display the contents of each template. Items are copied or deleted from the templates by selecting the item in the pane and clicking the appropriate button in the middle of the dialogue box. The Close button toggles to Open in order to allow the user to close templates and open different templates to display in the dialogue box.

11. If the file was previously open and then incorrectly closed, parts of the file may still be in RAM and the file is therefore still considered to be open. Windows considers the file to be in use, even though it does not appear to be open. When the user tries to open the file, the message indicates the file is still in use.

12. CTRL+F9

13. F11

14. Open the Browse by dialogue box and change the browse setting to Page instead of Field.

15. Insert the empty field, select the field, and then press CTRL+D and set the format of the field.

16. Insert the empty field using CTRL+F9. Move the insertion point inside the brackets and type a forward slash (/). Follow the slash with a note.

17. Page number, Date/Time, User Initials, Document Properties, Bookmarks and Cross-References, Comments

18. Create date because this date does not update or change when the document is opened on another day

19. ALT+F9

LESSON SEVEN

1. To automatically correct typos and spelling errors

2. To correct spelling errors, to correct typos, to quickly format awkward terms, to insert symbols, change the function of a key

3. Tools>AutoCorrect

4. Because AutoCorrect entries will always insert, so you will want to create a shortcut that will not be accidentally expanded (i.e., an actual word)

5. Open the AutoCorrect dialogue box, type a shortcut in the Replace box, and type the correct form in the With box.

6. Type and format the entry in the document itself. Carefully select the entry, avoiding paragraph marks and extra spaces (unless needed). Open the AutoCorrect dialogue box, check the Formatted entry box. Type a shortcut in the Replace box. Click OK.

7. Type the shortcut or the "replace" text and then press the Spacebar or any punctuation key.

8. In the Spelling and Grammar dialogue box, choose the correct word and click AutoCorrect. From the shortcut menu, choose AutoCorrect and then choose the correct word.

9. Press CTRL+Z as soon as the AutoCorrect entry inserts.

10. The Normal.dot and the *.ACL file.

11. AutoCorrect entries are available no matter what document or template you are using. AutoText entries can be separated into different template files so that they are only available when that template is in use. AutoCorrect entries will be changed by other AutoCorrect features such as automatic capitalization. AutoText entries are not subject to AutoCorrect features; they always maintain their formatting.

12. Type the text in a document and then select the text. Open the AutoText dialogue box (Tools>AutoCorrect>AutoText). Type a name for the entry and click Add. Or, type and select the entry. Press ALT+F3 to open the Create AutoText dialogue box. Type a name for the entry and press Enter.

13. Type the AutoText name (shortcut). When the fourth character of the AutoText name is typed, the suggestion box will appear. Press the Enter key. Or, type the AutoText name and press the F3 key.

14. Open a document based on the template that you want to use to store the AutoText entry. Open the AutoText dialogue box, change the Look in box to the specific template. Close the dialogue box. Select the text to be saved as an AutoText entry. Press ALT+F3. Name the AutoText entry and press Enter.

15. If an AutoText entry is created in the Default font, that entry can then be used in other documents where the default font is also defined, even though it may be different than the font used to create the AutoText entry. In this case, the AutoText entry will always insert into the document with the font of the surrounding text.

16. The Organizer

17. Open the AutoText dialogue box, select the entry and click Delete. The second way is to open the Organizer dialogue box and switch to the tab labeled AutoText. Select the entry or several entries and click Delete.

18. To combine a series of commands into a single command. Traditionally, macros have been used to save text, paragraphs, normals, and standard text, but this is best done using AutoText, AutoCorrect, or a text expander.

19. To open a document based on a template, to combine several editing commands into a single command, to automate a repetitive task.

20. Through the Tools menu: Tools, Macro, Record new macro, or double-click the REC button on the Status bar.

21. Macro names cannot contain spaces or punctuation.

22. Back up the template file that contains the Macros—most often the Normal.dot file.

23. AC (This shortcut would always be needed and there are no conflicts with other shortcuts or words.)

24. AT (Automatic capitalization will not override the formatting of an AutoText entry.)

25. AC (This shortcut would always be needed and there are no conflicts with other shortcuts or words.)

26. AT (Could not use AutoCorrect because this method would always insert an additional space after the nonbreaking space.)

27. AT (AutoCorrect would not be a good choice since "eat" is an actual word and might be expanded accidentally.)

28. Template (A template file would set up the formatting start to finish with no need to insert formatting as you type.)

29. AT in a specific template (Use AT to insert only when needed and only when using the template for that specific doctor/clinic.)

30. Macro (Macros are best for a series of commands.)

31. Macro (Macros are best for a series of commands.)

32. AT (Use AT to insert only when needed and only when using the template for that specific doctor/clinic.)

33. AC (This shortcut would always be needed since you would always want the misspelling to be corrected.)

34. AT or AC

35. AT (or third-party text expander). (AT entries are easier to manage than AutoCorrect and can be sorted into templates and shared with others.)

36. AT (AutoText entries maintain their formatting.)

LESSON EIGHT

1. Press F7 to open the Spelling and Grammar dialogue box; press ALT+F7 to select the next misspelled word and open the shortcut menu; click the ABC icon on the toolbar; choose Tools>Spelling and Grammar; or right-click on the misspelled word and choose the correct spelling from the shortcut menu.

2. The book with the X indicates the document still has spelling or grammar errors. The book with the check mark indicates the document has been corrected for spelling and grammar errors.

3. This command adds the selected word to the Custom dictionary so Word no longer marks it as incorrectly spelled.

4. The Main dictionary loads with Word (or Office) and serves as a reference for the spell check routine. Words not found in the Main dictionary are marked as incorrectly spelled. The Main dictionary cannot be edited, so new words are added to the Custom dictionary file. Word will also reference the Custom dictionary file to see if a word is incorrectly spelled.

5. If you notice immediately that you have added an incorrect word to the Custom dictionary, press CTRL+Z or click the Undo command. If you later realize a word needs to be removed from the list, go to Tools>Options>Spelling and Grammar. Click Dictionaries, then choose Edit (or Modify if using WordXP). Remove the word from the list.

6. Turn Spell check back on by opening the Spelling and Grammar dialogue box and placing the first check mark at Check spelling as you type.

7. Use the Formatting marks within the document combined with the toolbars and rulers, or use "What's This" by pressing Shift+F1 and clicking over the text in question.

8. Open a document based on a template containing the macro key assignments to be printed. Press CTRL+P to open the Print dialogue box. In the Print what box, choose Key Assignments.

9. Text is selected.

10. Home sends the insertion point to the beginning of a line.

    End sends the insertion point to the end of a line.

    CTRL+Home moves the insertion point to the beginning of a document.

    CTRL+End moves the insertion point to the end of a document.

11. ALT, F, C; CTRL+W; CTRL+F4; ALT+F4

12. F4

13. Shift+F5

14. Bold = CTRL+B

    Italic = CTRL+I

    Underline = CTRL+U

    Redo = CTRL+Y

    Change case = Shift+F3

    Open Save As dialogue box = CTRL+S or F12

    Font dialogue box = CTRL+D

15. F8 turns on Extend mode for selecting text. Press twice to select the word, press three times to select the sentence and four times to select the paragraph. Also, press F8 and then a character key and the text will be selected from the insertion point to the first occurrence of the character. Press Esc to turn off Extend mode or press a command key to apply the command and turn off Extend mode at the same time.

16. To remove a word or phrase just typed; to reverse a cut or paste; to undo the last action; to undo an AutoCorrect entry; to undo an automatic formatting change such as automatic numbering or automatic capitalization; to undo mistakes or random strikes on the keyboard.

17. Use the Find and Replace feature. Type the word in the "Find" box and leave the Replace box empty. Click Replace All.

18. Remove manual formatting from a paragraph.

19. Remove manual formatting from text.

20. Open the Find dialogue box.

21. Open the Find and Replace dialogue box.

22. Open the Go To dialogue box.

23. Change the View to Print Preview.

24. Decrease the font size by 1 point.

25. Format selected text as all caps.

26. Copy the formatting commands for the selected text.

27. Apply the copied formatting commands to the selected text.

28. Delete one word to the left.

29. Insert a manual page break.

30. Move to the beginning of the previous paragraph.

31. Removes the selection from the text and places the insertion point at the beginning (left arrow) or the end (right arrow) of the selected text

32. Pressing the Shift key along with the navigation keys will select the text as the insertion point moves from its original position to the position designated by the navigation key.

33. Go to Tools>Options>Spelling and Grammar (or right-click on the Spelling and Grammar icon on the Status bar and choose Options). In the dialogue box, click the Settings button. Remove check marks at the various options so Word will no longer mark that type of potential error.

LESSON NINE

1. Key assignments, toolbars, icons, menus, shortcut menus

2. Right-click over any toolbar and choose Customize; go to Tools>Customize; or double-click (left mouse) in a blank area around the toolbars.

3. The Customize dialogue box

4. On the Customize dialogue box, under the Commands tab

5. Hold down the ALT key while dragging the icon from its original position to a new position on the same toolbar or a different toolbar.

6. Hold down the CTRL key and the ALT key while dragging the icon from its original position to a new toolbar.

7. The & (ampersand)

8. Open the Customize dialogue box and click the Keyboard button in the bottom right corner.

9. ALT pressed alone activates the Menu bar and the Title bar. The ALT key pressed along with another key invokes a specific command assigned to that key combination.

10. ALT or CTRL

11. Toolbar tab, New button

12. The Commands tab, under the Category New menu

LESSON TEN

Answers to the Problem Solving questions can be found on the following pages:

1. p. 68

2. p. 61

3. p. 140

4. p. 143

5. p. 73

6. p. 158

7. p. 113

8. p. 177

9. p. 175

10. p. 162

11. p. 135

12. p. 249

13. p. 35
14. p. 23
15. p. 23
16. p. 35
17. p. 248
18. p. 155
19. p. 245
20. p. 183
21. p. 35
22. p. 117
23. p. 41
24. p. 187
25. p. 181
26. p. 49
27. p. 148
28. p. 225